Constant Antoine Roux

Dietetic Nutrition, Growth and Sport

Constant Antoine Roux

Dietetic Nutrition, Growth and Sport

ScienciaScripts

Imprint

Any brand names and product names mentioned in this book are subject to trademark, brand or patent protection and are trademarks or registered trademarks of their respective holders. The use of brand names, product names, common names, trade names, product descriptions etc. even without a particular marking in this work is in no way to be construed to mean that such names may be regarded as unrestricted in respect of trademark and brand protection legislation and could thus be used by anyone.

Cover image: www.ingimage.com

This book is a translation from the original published under ISBN 978-620-2-26838-7.

Publisher:
Sciencia Scripts
is a trademark of
Dodo Books Indian Ocean Ltd. and OmniScriptum S.R.L publishing group

120 High Road, East Finchley, London, N2 9ED, United Kingdom
Str. Armeneasca 28/1, office 1, Chisinau MD-2012, Republic of Moldova, Europe
Printed at: see last page
ISBN: 978-620-5-75846-5

Summary

DIETETIC NUTRITION AND AFRICAN SPECIFICITIES

Continental Francophone Course

Sports medicine

IOC/ACNOA/CNO-CIV

Abidjan 27-29 JUNE 2012

Ivory Coast

Professor Constant Antoine ROUX .

NUTRITION-DIETETICS WHY?

NUTRITION-DIETETICS WHY to IMPROVE Performance.

Food requires two necessities:

1)- BIO-ENERGETIC needs to maintain the activity

-      of life

-      muscle.

2)-Plastic needs

including: -protection

-repair} of tissues

-- modelling

NUTRITION-DIETETICS AND AFRICAN SPECIFICITIES

The man for his survival spends

For growth

For the renewal of cells, organelles and molecules

For maintenance

For physical exercise

The man spends what?

Nutrients

Assimilable molecules

Ensuring the synthesis and renewal

Energy sources

I-/-ENERGY NEEDS.

A-Quantitative aspects

Average caloric.of the athlete-loss of the organism during the effort -

basic expenditure: 40cal/h/m2

The expenses due to THERMOREGULATION increase by 5% when the temperature decreases by 10°c!

Data from Kester and Knipping:

Physical activities - Caloric needs/hr.

Soccer; rugby; handball;

rowing; tennis; jumping; } 300 â 500 cal.

cycling.

Marathon; fencing;

boxing; swimming(speed);} 500 â 700 cal.

figure skating;

basketball; water polo.

Running (long distance); wrestling:

Cross-country skiing;tennis(-single). } 700â 900 cal.

Data from Kester and Knipping

-Physical activities Caloric requirements/hr

Running (½ distance); skiing (speed). } 900 cal.

B--Qualitative aspects.

Necessity of a balanced distribution between several constituents-

1-Carbohydrates (liver; muscles) = 55% total calories = 1g = 4cal.

2- LIPIDS (Animals; plants) .

= 30% total calories = 1 g = 9 cal

3- PROTEINS

= 15% total calories = 1 g = 4 cal.

II - /- PLASTIC NEEDS

Contributed by food:

-    essential to life.

-    cannot be produced by the organism.

1-Nitrogenic requirements . - Essential Amino Acids .

2- Vitamin requirements : (2 TYPES)

a-) -Those with a real analeptic action:

-    Vitamin B complex

(vit. B1 ; B6)

-    Vitamin C.

b-)-Liposolubles .

3- Hydromineral needs (liquid entry and exit)

-    Water: each calorie ingested is accompanied by 1 g of water

-    food provides ½ water.

<u>"It is necessary to DRINK without thirst.</u>

-       Mineral salts: in vegetables and fruits.

There are three types of RATION.

- 1- ation of Training .

- 2- Competition Ration.

- 3- Recovery Ration.

1- TRAINING Ration.

- No particular dietary constraints!

- MEALS REQUIRED: - Sufficient quantity.

- Varies. - Balances!

1 1- Training meal,

Requires Q 4 daily meals:

1-a)-- Breakfast brings 25% of the ration-

2-b)-- Breakfast : 35 %- of the ration .

3-c)-- Gouter : 15% of the ration .

4-d)-- Dinner (evening meal) : 25 % of the ration-

DRINK: Throughout the day, at meal times. "DRINK WITHOUT THIRST"! ! !

2 - COMPETITION RATION.

3 HOURS LAW!!! -

the last meal should be taken three

3 3) hours before the competition.

WAIT RATION: ¼ â 1/8 fat, water + 10 g glucose.

- - every ½ hour or hour.

- - last intake : ½ hour before the competition.

3-Ration of RECUPERATION and PER-COMPETITIVE.

- Complete HYDRATATION.

-Recharge carbohydrate reserves +++.

- From the beginning of the warm-up:

Start DRINKING.

Collective team (soccer), DRINK as much as possible during the warm-up.

- - The diet must be adapted to the individual.

pleasant to the taste (palatable).

-The proportions of the diet depend:

duration of effort,

of its intensity,

the eating habits of the athlete, the degree of training.

- a trained athlete uses preferably his LIPIDS : he saves his carbohydrate stocks.

Two key concepts:

You must:

" DRINKING WITHOUT THIRST."

"Prescribe, as in prescription,

PHYSICAL ACTIVITY

(30mn or 3 times :10mn/day)

Tribute

to Dr. Thianar NDOYE

(nutritionist - dietician - helas , â la retrăite , in Senegal de Rufisque).

AFRICAN DIETETICS

Is there a specificity of African Dietetic Nutrition?

Sport is part of the pure African tradition: example of wrestling in the Sahel where the diet of the village champion is a matter for all.

Dietetics is essential for growth!

- In Europe, in 50% of the medical anomalies encountered in young athletes, 15% are related to nutritional deficiencies.

- In Africa, this percentage remains higher (protein-calorie malnutrition).

Nutritionists define three types of needs:

1-the energy needs ,

2-   plastic needs ,

3-   maintenance and protection.

The energy is produced by

Carbohydrates,

Lipids and

Protein -

Plastic is provided by

Protein (animal or vegetable)

Maintenance and Protection are provided by

Vitamins and minerals.

There are interferences between them and with carbohydrates, lipids and proteins.

In sportsmen, the pre and per-competitive rations must only privilege the support of glycemia, by the drink, the rehydration, the ressucration, the mineralization, the alkalization of the sportsman.

"ONE MUST DRINK WITHOUT THIRST".

There IS a Tropical Sports Dietetics, singularly African, made of its own specificity and a variant of adaptation based on the horizontal typology L.T.C. (Legumes - Tubers - Cereals).

Nutritional Profiles of Dietetic Nutrition in Africa :- WHO Factsheets

4-   Profile types: A/-SAHELIAN-B/-FORESTIER-COTIER-C/- UGANDA -D/- MAGHREBIAN

Net Protein Utilization Index (N.P.U.)

Dominant Culinary Association .

Nutritional profiles of dietetic nutrition in Africa

Type reference MAURITANIA : C.L.T.

C 52 L5 T 0.3-Total =57.3% of total ration. - Most economical profile !!!

A-/-SAHELIEN - Reference Senegal : C.L.T.

C52 L15 T6 -Total = 73% of total ration

B-/-FORESTIER - COTIER -Group BURKINA-FASO, MALI : C.L.T.---C75 L12 T3-Total =90%   of total ration .

Forestry type -Wood : Group IVORY COAST, BENIN, TOGO, CAMEROON : C.T.L.---C46 T40 L8-Total = 94 % of the total ration.

C: UGANDA - Group GABON, CAR, DRC ---T.C.L. -T64 C14 L7 - Total=85% of total ration .

NUTRITION DIÉTÉTIQUE SPÉCIFICTÉ AFRICAINE

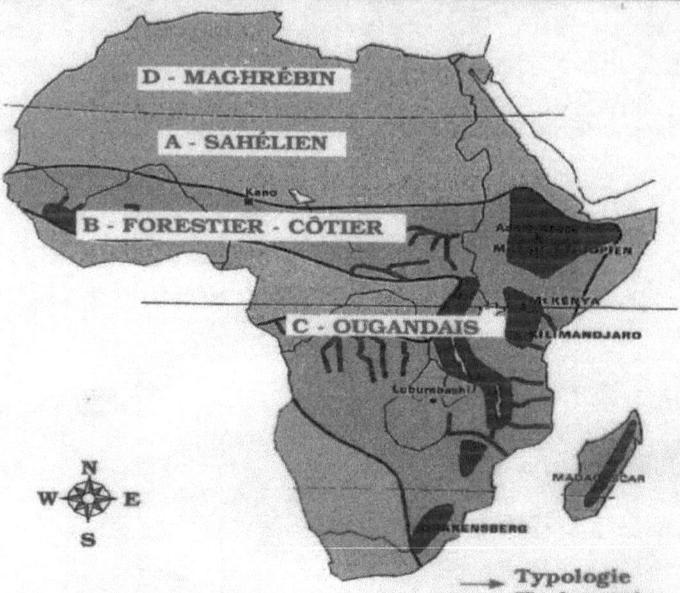

→ Typologie Horizontale

Fiche Signalitique O.M.S.
- . Légumineuses
- . Tubercules
- . Céréales

4 Types de Profil
- A. SAHÉLIEN
- B. FORESTIER - CÔTIER
- C. OUGANDAIS
- D. MAGHRÊBIEN

*** Indice Utilisation Protéinique Nette (U.P.N.)**
*** Associations Culinaires Dominantes**
Structures de la consommation

Growth and sports: the growth plate (cc)

<< sport and the child: traumas of the growth plate .

By Professor **Roux** Constant Antoine;

Sport and children: growth plate injuries

Introduction

In children, sport is an indispensable element, essential because it promotes :

- his psychomotor development and social learning ;

- Body awareness;

- his learning of the gesture ;

- the concept of training;

- respect for the rules of life, for others

- the opponent of the same age, and the referee.

Three (03) types of problems must be taken into account:

1. growth (the growth plate)

2. Sport (stimulates growth)

The stressful physical exercise (young gymnasts...), associated with an unbalanced diet leads to a delay in the onset of puberty by 2 to 3 years:

- absence of menstruation due to lack of restrogen; amenorrhea causing a loss of 5% per year of bone mass, identical to that of menopausal women.

- poor bone development;

3. energy expenditure (muscle development, tendon elasticity, ease of metabolic adaptation). *More than 20 %* compared to the adult.

IN THE CHILD

Fractures are different because the child's skeleton has an increasing plasticity. The sequels are never definitive:

- growth is capable of the best and the worst

- it can reshape or amplify everything!

- **The evaluation of fractures in children is subject to two errors:**

--The **first** error is to consider that the child is an adult in miniature, and therefore to project the experience of adult orthopedics into the estimation of these fractures.

--The **second** error is to reduce everything to an old aphorism that is unfortunately all too common: <<**growth fixes everything**! >> In reality, in order to judge objectively a child's fracture, two situations must be differentiated:

1. fractures affecting the extremity of a long bone: these fractures are always serious, because they affect the **growth plate,** and call into question the morphology, the length, the articular congruence.

2. fractures that affect the diaphyseal areas: they are all generally **benign** and heal faster the younger the child.

Diaphyseal angulations usually straighten with growth; only rotational anomalies, resulting from poorly conducted orthopedic treatment, are definitive.

There is therefore everything to fear from an epiphyseal fracture and everything to hope for from a diaphyseal fracture!

To understand the evolutionary future of a fracture in children, and consequently the sequelae, it is necessary to define the **growth** plate: it holds the morphological future of the bone.

Macroscopically:

It is a more or less linear structure, **invisible to the** standard radiographic study,

MACROSCOPY (DIAGRAM AND RADIOGRAPHY) OF THE GROWTH PLATE

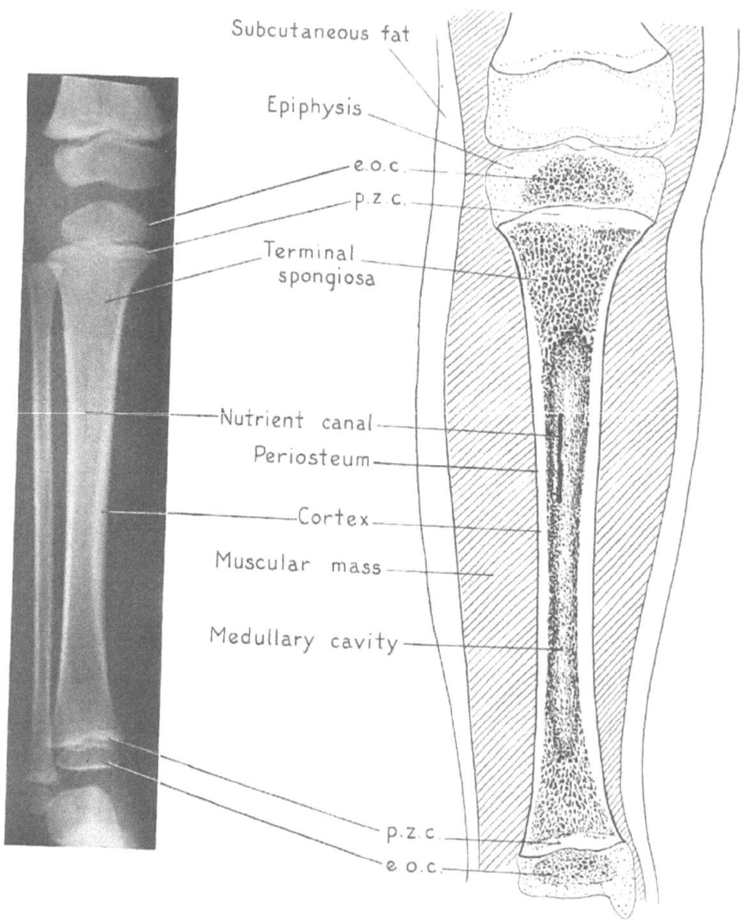

Transparent" "invisible" linear structure that can be clearly seen in the adolescent, between the epiphysis and the metaphysis of a long bone (cfrt.longitudinal section of a growth plate according to Siffert and Gilbert.)

<u>**Microscopically:**</u>

The histological study provides us with valuable information. **The growth plate.**

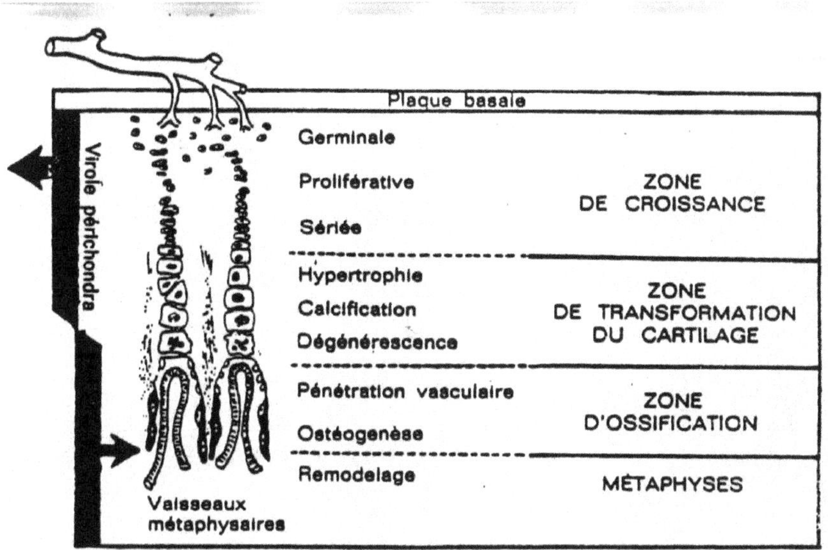

Longitudinal section of a growth plate (Siffert and Gilbert)

It individualizes, from the pole to the equator of a basic model, **4 main layers** of cells embedded in an intercellular substance, capped by a layer of epiphyseal bone tissue: *the basal plate.*

I. <u>**first layer of cells: the germinative layer,**</u>

Consists of small cells, little differentiated, scattered in a dense intercellular substance.

II. <u>**second layer of cells: the serial layer .**</u>

Thicker than the previous one, so called because the cells are arranged in parallel longitudinal columns, it is the true germinal layer of the cartilage, **the engine of growth.**

The cell is the seat of many cellular multiplications; *all the mitoses are synchronous* at the same level. In the cells we observe:

- an increase in granular endoplasmic reticulum;

- hypertrophy of the golgi apparatus.

- they are surrounded by their secretion: the intercellular substance. Composed of: *collagen fibers*, *proteoglycans* (e.g. M.P.S.: chondroitin sulfate; hyaluronic acid), structural *glycoproteins*; *lipids*; *water* and *mineral salts*.

The weft where the hydroxy-apatite crystals will be fixed, is built on the collagen framework. **It is a very solid zone** thanks to the density of these fibrillar elements.

III. **Third layer: the hypertrophic layer.**

Thicker and **more fragile**, by proportional reduction of the intercellular fundamental substance._The cell does not multiply any more, does not secrete any more intercellular fundamental substance.

It hypertrophies and shows :

a. *signs of preparation for calcification*, with the appearance of : - dense granules in the mitochondria, -vesicles in the plasma membrane. Correlatively, the fundamental substance becomes mature and prepares for calcification.

b. *modification of the collagen* which polymerizes with destruction of the proteoglycans.

c. *the phospholipid vesicles* are preparing to *burst and release the calcium.*

N.b. It is precisely between the cartilage transformation zone and the ossification zone that the

The ring or **the perichondral ring of Chung:** Zone where the **fractures of the growth cartilage** are located.

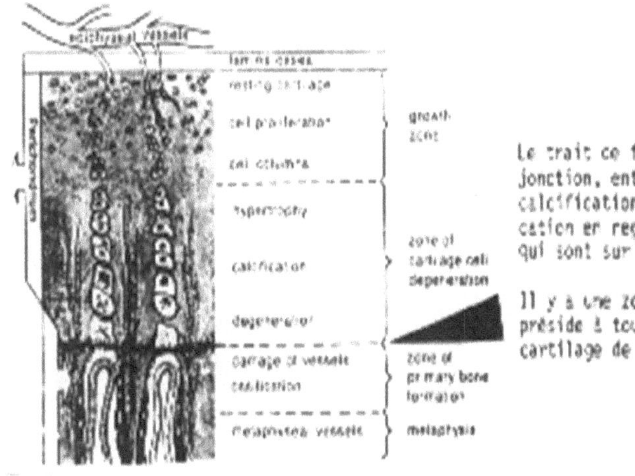

Fracture location: perichondral ring weakness zone

IV. <u>fourth layer the degenerative layer.</u>

It is a thin layer, it has no function of its own, and there is a ***death of*** the chondrocyte due to the disappearance of exchanges, concomitant with ***a calcification of*** the intercellular fundamental substance in contact,

Constituent: **the calcification front of the growth plate.**

For many, **growth plate is** a histological structure interposed between the epiphysis and the diaphysis, the **bone <u>responsible for </u>the growth in length of a long bone.**

This definition, although classic, is inaccurate, because it is too restrictive!

It is important to know that at the end of a long bone, such as the humerus or the femur,

There are actually **several growth plates**:

1.   some contribute to ***the growth in length of the bone***, *this is* the role reserved for the **conjugation cartilage.**

2.   the others, which are located **in the epiphyses or apophyses,** contribute to

perfecting the morphology of the bone, giving it its congruence, its anatomical identity.

Whatever the topography of these cartilages, whatever their morphology (they can be circular or roughly rectangular), all have the same histological structure.

Within the same bone, all cartilages are integrated in a perfectly synchronized game and the damage of a single cartilage by a **trauma** is likely to disrupt the harmony of the whole system and to question the morphological future of the bone.

Thus, **six growth plates** participate in the development of a bone:

- 4 for the *upper* extremity

- 2 for the *lower* end

Femur: <u>**4 c.c. For the upper extremity**</u> :

- conjugation cartilage

- epiphyseal growth plate

- 1 - **apophyseal** cartilage for the ***greater trochanter***

- **apophyseal** cartilage for the ***lesser trochanter.***

The growth plate.

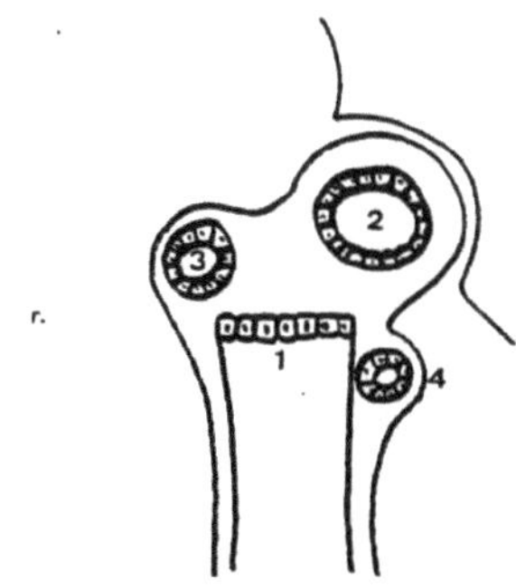

Circular morphology	Upper end of the femur

Upper extremity of the femur: Femur: 2 cc.

- 1 conjugation cartilage for *length growth*

- 1 *epiphyseal growth* plate (circular morphology)

Thus, a common fracture of the **greater trochanter** can cause a **coxa valga**, disorganizing the relationships between the growth plates.

Similarly, damage to the conjugation cartilage of the **upper extremity of the femur** is always serious (30% of the growth in length of the femur).

The femur measures *15 cm at* birth and *45 cm* at the end of growth. This cartilage has 10 cm of growth in length.

A *fracture of the femoral neck* leads to a shortening that is all the more severe, the more important the *younger the athlete is in bone age.*

On the other hand: the damage of the conjugation cartilage of *the lower extremity of the femur* is **more serious because** it holds 70% of the growth in length of the bone (potential quantifiable at 70% of 30 cm: 20 cm!!!).

The growth plate.

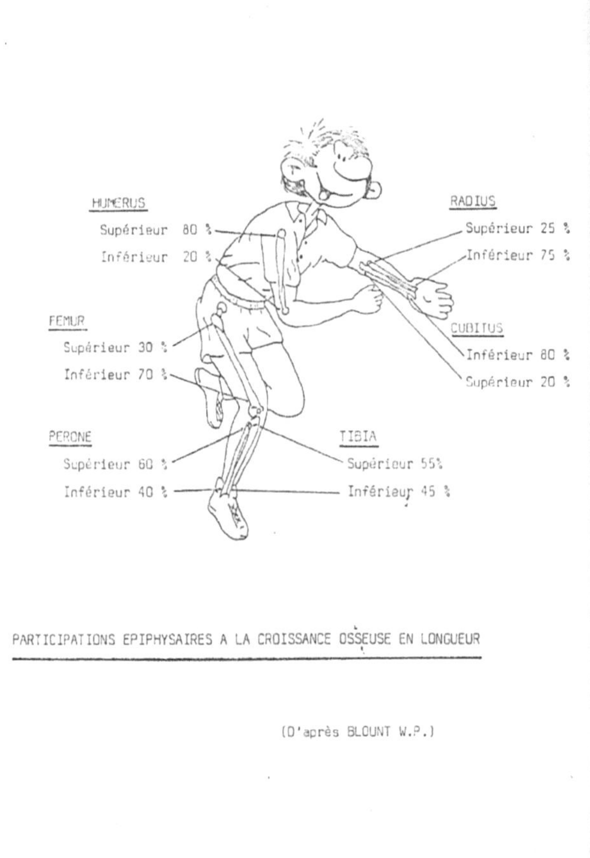

PARTICIPATIONS EPIPHYSAIRES A LA CROISSANCE OSSEUSE EN LONGUEUR

(D'après BLOUNT W.P.)

>   Referring to the **longitudinal growth section according to Siffert & Gilbert**:

>   On either side of the growth plate, **metaphysis** (top) and **epiphysis** (bottom) *arrive and depart from the*

>   **vessels** that *will*

S feed it,

S vascularize it.

In the young, a shock, trauma against the knee joint of the growth plate → growth disorders of this cartilage (*have ă in mind the diagram of Blount W.P.with percentage of epiphyseal participation ă the bone growth in length*) .

Aphorism:<Far from **the elbow, near the knee, be careful with the shoulder, without forgetting the wrist.**>

Growth rate:

Lower extremity of the femur: 70%.

Upper extremity of the tibia: 55%.

Upper extremity of the perone: 60% (***near the knee***)

S Superior extremity of the humerus: 80% (***be careful with the*** shoulder)

S Lower extremity of the ***ulna: 80% (not forgetting the*** wrist*)*

S Lower extremity of the radius: 75% (***including the*** wrist)

In sports medicine for young athletes, it is **imperative** to :

>   **not to be unaware of** the *classification of* **Salter and Harris** who classified the traumatisms of the growth plates in:

>   *five (05) types*

THE GROWTH CHART

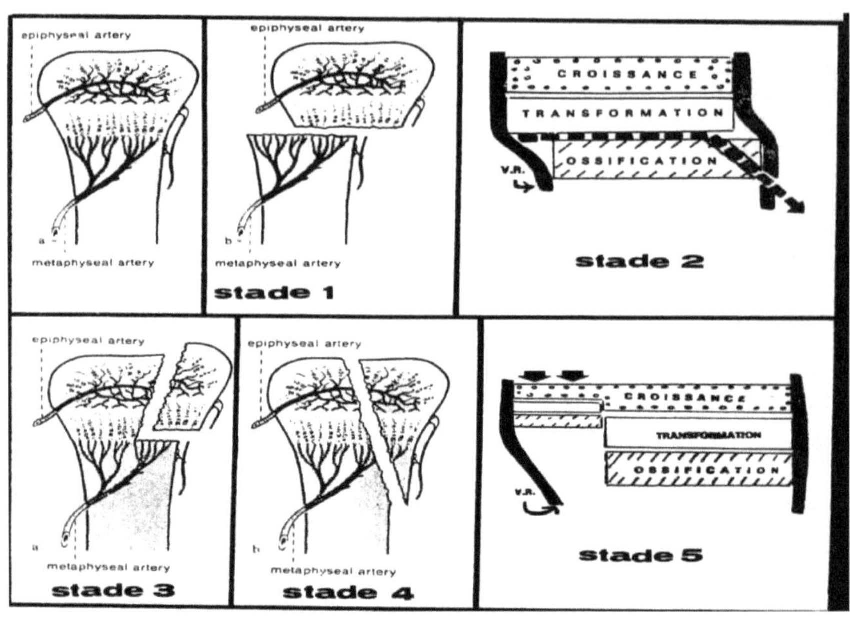

epiphyseal artery
metaphyseal artery
stade 1
epiphyseal artery
metaphyseal artery
CROISSANCE
TRANSFORMATION
OSSIFICATION
V.R.
stade 2
epiphyseal artery
metaphyseal artery
stade 3
epiphyseal artery
metaphyseal artery
stade 4
CROISSANCE
TRANSFORMATION
OSSIFICATION
V.R.
stade 5

Mechanism of trauma (Salter and Harris)

<u>Salter and Harris *Type I*:</u>

S The **most trivial**

S pure *epiphyseal detachment*

- **Reduction must be perfect**

- *Generally excellent prognosis*

(the germinal cells of the growth plate are intact).

<u>Salter and Harris Type II:</u>

- More or less serious, *it is most frequent*

- **The *fracture line passes* through the entire *growth plate* at one end where it rises and detaches a *metaphyseal corner***

- **Easy early reduction**

- **Generally good prognosis**

<u>Salter and Harris Type III</u>:

- **Severe** (the **very type of intra-articular fracture** separating the epiphysis in two)

- Epiphyseal detachment in the growth plate

- Anatomical reduction + associated internal restraint (pin)

- *Prognosis reserve*

<u>Salter and Harris Type IV</u>:

- **Very serious: articular fracture** with an oblique line that separates the epiphysis and the metaphysis in a corner

- **Crosses the growth plate** which is epiphyseal-metaphyseal

- Imposes a perfect anatomical reduction (possibly surgical)

- **Poor prognosis**

<u>**Salter and Harris type V**</u>:

- **The most fearsome**

- Crushing of the growth plate by compression

- **Prognosis always serious**

-Possible association type I,II,III or IV with a type V

- This fracture ***often goes unnoticed*** and escapes radiological investigations

- ***Diagnosis often made only at the stage of sequelae***

- <u>**In conclusion**</u>: we **must differentiate between two types of fracture lines**:

- -the **horizontal** lines

- -the **vertical** lines

- it is necessary to differentiate between **two types** of *fracture lines*:

- -1_**horizontal** lines of **the s.c.**: generally a <u>**good prognosis**</u>

- -2_**Vertical** lines **of the c.c.: are serious** because they expose to the shift.

C.C. TRAUMATISM

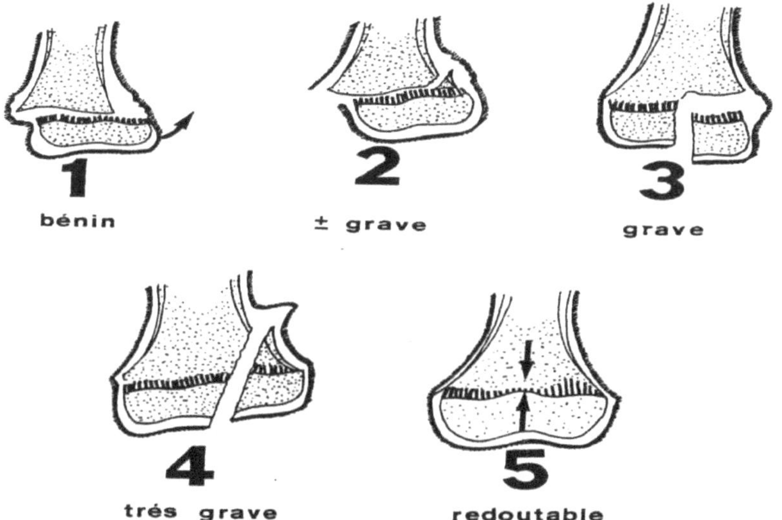

Classification of Salter and Harris (J.Bone and Joint Surg. 1963, 45 A: 587)

Behind a trauma, can **be hidden a type V diagnosis,** characterized by

- ✓ **a deviation of axis or**

- ✓ **a shortening of the limb**, *harmful* consequences *for the young person's sports career*

SOME RULES OF PREVENTION:

<u>**For the young athlete**</u>

Sports practice in children: **three periods to respect**

- **5-12 years**: from school to puberty

- **From 11 to 15 years old**: pre-puberty period

- **From 15 years**: end of adolescence

<u>**PREVENTION: Three periods**</u>

❖ **1-From 5 to 12 years:**

(from school to puberty): **Introductory sports** :

> The child plays as long as he wants to.

> No pressure to go beyond his desires. ***Recommended sports***: **Gymnastics; Swimming.**

> Prevention: Three periods.

> 2 /-From 11 to 15 years: Pre-puberty period. -**Acceleration of somatic growth. Competitive sport -Allowed** in the same age category -Advised!

> <u>Pre-puberty period</u>

> Moral <u>education </u>and preparation for future life in society: respect for others, the most effective. **Do not perform <u>resistance </u>tests!**

- <u>**Prevention: Three periods**</u>.

> -3--)-After 15 years old! ***<u>End of adolescence.</u>***

I **Allow** training, muscularity and progressive resistance tests,

J -- **without fear of disrupting growth.**

-- ***In training period*** :

J *1-Fostering* SPORTS-EDUCATED designs.

J ***2-Avoid*** overtraining:

Prevention:

J   *--in **training period**:*

J - 3-Take into account the sacred time of the **COMPENSATIVE REST**!

J - 4--It is necessary to **associate sports with opposite effects**

J Gymnastics / Running .

J Tennis-Swimming / Hand Sports - Cycling .

- **The NEEDS of the Young Athlete are:**

a)   **Those of the growth**

b)   **Those specific to the sport practiced**

- **Physiologically:**

\>   **low storage capacity of carbohydrate reserves of the young**

\>   **it is: --more explosive, fast, --less enduring .**

\>   **- Before puberty:**

-    **- high risk of *hypoglycemia***

-    ***- Inability* to *produce lactates***

-    ***- Unable to* excel *in sprinting***

- **For the child:**

- **It is necessary to take into account**

- **its development** →

S **Adapt practice rules to the child's physiology.**

-- It is important:

S **1) to make him practice:**

- **A *complementary sport* (swimming, athletics)**

- **An *individual and team sport***

- **For the child**:

It is important:

-- 2) to associate:

- An ***indoor activity***

- An outdoor ***sport***

- - sports that require the spine cannot be completed (horse riding, judo)

- **Prevention:**

<u>from a **physiological and mental point of view**</u>

Every child is different in terms of

S to his answer and

S to its tolerance to effort

- due to variations in *growth **rate**,* anthropometric indices, **gender** and ***health status***

- Recommendation of the **Council of Europe:**

- **Age of the beginning of the competition**: **16 years old** !!! (closing of the c.c.)

- -Closure of the growth plate:

- Gargon: **16-17** years old

- Girl: **14** years old

- **In High Competition,**

- Know how to **protect the young athlete**:

- **Medical certificate required**

- **Minimum supervision** *three times* **during the sports season (1- at the beginning: certificate of aptitude, license; 2- in the middle: the treve; 3- at the end: assessment)**

- **Comply with the rigors of** the *upgrade certificate*

The OVERCLASSIFICATION CERTIFICATE

The athletes are classified in 5 categories:

- **Senior**

- **Junior**

- **Cadet**

- **Minimal**

- **Benjamin and Chick**

categories	boys	girls	From
Seniors	19 years old	18 years old	
Juniors	17 years old	16 years old	1st year
	18 years old	17 years old	2nd year
Cadets	15 years old	14 years old	1st year
	16 years old	15 years old	2nd year
Minimes	14 years old	13 years old	1st year
	15 years old	14 years old	2nd year
benjamins	12 years old		

- **<u>DOUBLE OVERCLASSIFICATION</u> simple:**

■ **Absence of albumin**

- **Ruffier robustness index (A-B) > 8**

- **<u>CV x 100</u> > 6 P = pulse**

P

- **Total absence of any pathological antecedent**

- **Tuberculin reaction: -- Positive for more than 6 months**

--Negative less than 10 days

■ **2nd year upgrade certificate valid for 120 days**

■ **DOUBLE OVERCLASSING 1st YEAR is FORMALLY PROHIBITED!!!**

- **When, in spite of everything**, **cartilage trauma occurs,** in young athletes, it is a

<u>**THERAPEUTIC EMERGENCY!!!**</u>

THERAPEUTIC METHODS:

They are **double:**

- **Preventive**

- **curative**

<u>A -**PREVENTIVE METHODS**</u>

Childhood trauma is *often <u>overlooked</u>*

Difference between:

- diaphyseal fractures (good prognosis)

- Epiphyseal detachment

- The adage *"Growth will correct the residual deformation*

  - ✓ acceptable for angulations and

  - ✓ moderate shortening of the **diaphysis**

  - ✓ **At the level of the**

- cartilage and epiphysis, there is <u>only room for </u>rigorous and meticulous reduction

In epiphyseal detachment fractures

it is necessary to require from

- *very good X-ray pictures*: the *cost of the fee is too high*

- **Early diagnosis is crucial**

- Obvious for big trips

- Difficult for small movements, during pure detachment.

To do so:

- We **can't tolerate bad X-ray pictures**

- Do not hesitate to use *tomographic* examination*, Arthro-Scan, MRI*

- *Look for the smallest metaphyseal fragment*, signature of the trauma

(sign of THURSTON and POLAND)

- **Study of the cliches:** *carefully* **thought out**

it is on it that the therapeutic conduct depends:

Reduction - orthopedic

-surgical

A decision of great consequence:

growth is at stake

- **Orthopedic method:**

Urgent realization

With minuție, under radiological control

because recent trauma = easy reduction

it's a matter of time

- **Orthopedic method:**

Any reduction must be maintained by **external and internal restraint**: **percutaneous pinning** from epiphysis to metaphysis with support on the opposite diaphyseal cortex (take care of the peripheral structures)

- **Surgical method**

the indication of a bloody route (often the case in types III and IV) requires the scrupulous respect of certain rules:

- ***Deperiostage to be avoided***

- ***Gentle, careful but anatomical reduction***

- ***Restraint*** either by pin

often by screw or screwed plate

totally sparing the growth plate

- **These two therapeutic methods, orthopedic and surgical, require a *plaster-post-operative contention,* more or less long depending on the epiphyses.**

B -<u>THERAPEUTIC</u> METHODS

always preceded by a prognosis of growth with:

J - measurement

- bone age

- - (using the *Green Anderson* and *Blount* tables)

<u>indications</u>:-- epiphysiodesis sequelae

- -imperfection of reduction

<u>**THERAPEUTIC METHODS**</u>

They are interested in:

1 -- **Growth disorders**

2 - **Axial deviations.**

1--Growth disorders:

-total epiphysiodesis no longer allows for growth restoration

-their treatment requires *surgery (legalization* involving either:

- Lying down on the traumatized limb

- Shortening or even stoppage of growth on the opposite side

2 --Axial deviations:

Once diagnosed ^must be treated because their **aggravation is progressive *until the end of growth*** (compromising -stopp- the sporting future of the young)

-2 types of surgical action:

- Osteotomy

- desepiphysiodese

- **2--Axial deviations**

2 -a) -Correction of deviation by ***osteotomy*** on the metaphyseal bone side ^ straightening and correction of angulation

---***final*** if performed ***at the end of growth***

---**temporary** if performed before (growth plate remains) .

2-- Axial deviations

■ 2-b) By ***desepiphysiodese*** (work of Langenskiold and Bright) this intervention necessitates:

-50% of intact cartilage (ensuring growth resumption)

-Complete atraumatic lifting of ***the epiphysiodesis bridge*** (identification and analysis by mapping of the remaining growth plate)

GENERAL CONCLUSION

GROWTH and SPORTS

ERROR BY EXCES !

ERROR BY DEFAULT!

- The odds of childhood fractures are often wrongly sized.

Before assessing a child's fracture, **one question must be answered**:

Was there or was there not damage to the growth plate?

> In the shadow of the ossified nuclei are hidden **growth plates** that can react surreptitiously

Judging a fracture in a young athlete means placing the trauma in a trajectory defined by three coordinates:

- The **growth time** that has been consumed

- The growth time left to go

- The future of sports ?

- Stiffness after one year is definitive

- Don't expect too much from secondary arthrolysis

- Behind a seemingly benign trauma, a Salter-Harris type V may be hidden, a source of desaxation and shortening

- Orthopedic, school and sports injuries

- Extraordinary functional rehabilitation of young athletes with anatomical lesions

This is not an excuse

Functional adaptation masks the disability but does not eliminate it

■ Loss of pronosupination, compensated by shoulder movements.

Hip stiffness, compatible with real sports activity.

■ Elbow movements can be normal, despite a valgus ulna

■ A shortening of the femur → oblique pelvis and low back pain An ulna-valgus can lead to secondary ulnar palsy.

CONCLUSION

■ The training and the practice of the sport must be done in the **same category of physiological age**

■ Beware of **abusive upgrading** and **double upgrading**!

■ Beware of overtraining! (pubalgia, OSGOOD- SCHLATTER disease).

■ **Yes** to **compensatory rest**!

■ Yes to a well-balanced nutrition-dietetics

CONCLUSION and PREVENTION

- **Always warn the family of a *possible disorder* before the end of the growth!**

- Prevention is the best medicine!

Preventing growth plate injuries in young athletes ??? **It is the extremity of the bone that holds the future of the fractures of the child athlete IT IS NECESSARY TO AVOID CUTTING THE PINK BUTTON!**

(avoid to ruin the rose in the bud!)

- The 9 th AFRICAN GAMES

have already started

- The 2nd AFRO-ASIATIC GAMES

are at our doors, here in ALGIERS

- **Friends ,Sports Physicians**

GOOD GAMES to you all

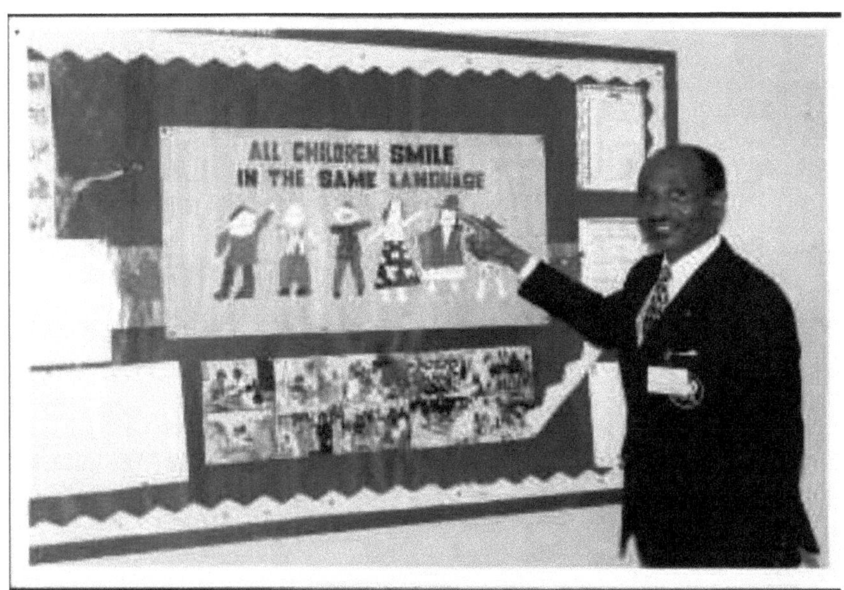

All children smile in the same language

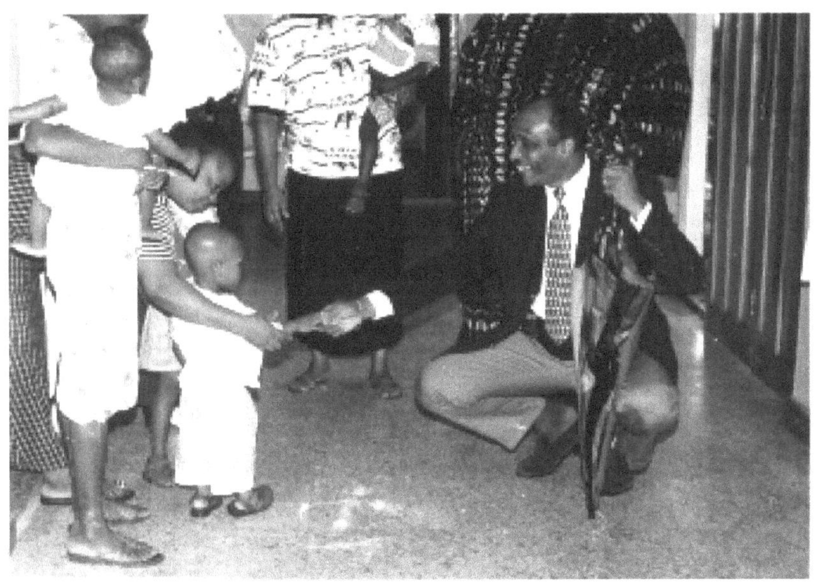

Bibliography:

1.   Aitken.A. P.: *Fractures of the ep/physes*.Clin.Orthop.41:19.1965.

2.   Blount, W.P. *Fractures in Children* (Baltimore: The Williams & Wilkins Company, 1955)

3.   Dimeglio *A.-la Cro/ssance en orthopedie -Sauramps* Medical Diffusion Vigot 1987.

4.   Dimeglio A. *Orthopedie Pediatrique quotidienne* --Sauramps Medical - Diffusion Vigot 1991

5.   Green W.T ,Wyatt G.M. and Anderson M.*Orthoroentgenography as a method measuring the bones extremities*(J.Bone Joint Surg, 1946,28,60-65.)

6.   Laurence G.-Orthopedie du premier âge -les Cahiers Bailliere 2nd edition-1966

7.   Masse P. and Taussig G. *Inegalities of length of the lower limbs in children* --les Cahiers Bailliere -1978

8.   Micheli.L.*The Young Athlete,in Sports Medicine and Physiology*.W.B.Saunders Company Chap18)

9.   Pous J.G, Dimeglio A.et Goalard J.A et C.-the *growing hip - Orthopedic problems* -Les Cahiers Bailliere -1976

10.   Rang.M.Children's *Fractures*(Philadelphia and Toronto J.B.Lippincott Company,1974)

11.   Salter R.B.and Harris W.R.-Injuriesinvolvingthe *epiphyseal plate* J.: (J. Bone and Joint Surg 45-A-587-622,1963)

12.   Sperryn Peter N. *Sport and Medicine* -Butterworths-London-1983

13.   Tachdjian M.:*Pediatric Orthopaedics*(Philadelphia W.B.Saunders Company,1972)

14.   Roux .C.A *-Course continental Francophone Medecine du Sport IOC/ACNOA/CNO-CIV Abidjan 27-29 June 2012*

15.   Sperryn Peter N: *Sport medicine -Diet 69-79* -Butterworths London -1983

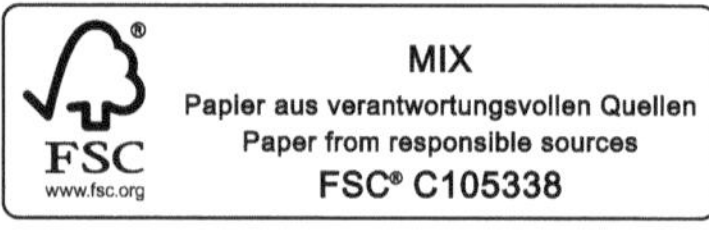

Printed by Books on Demand GmbH, Norderstedt / Germany